JUICING FOR DIVERTICULITIS

A 1000-Day Healthy Diet Cookbook for Beginners with Gut-Friendly, Anti-Inflammatory Fruit and Vegetable Blend Recipes.

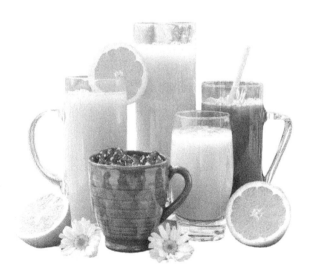

AVELINE WINTER

TABLE OF CONTENT

INTRODUCTION

Have you ever wondered if a glass of vibrant, nutrient-packed juice could be the key to soothing the discomfort of diverticulitis? Welcome to *"Juicing for Diverticulitis"* by Aveline Winter – your comprehensive guide to harnessing the power of juicing for digestive well-being.

As we know, the world is filled with endless health trends, juicing remains a timeless practice celebrated for its numerous benefits. Join me as we discover how juicing can be a flavorful remedy for those navigating the challenges of diverticulitis.

Within these pages, you'll find a lot of information aimed at making your juicing experience both enjoyable and health-conscious. It contains detailed ingredients, each chosen with care to support digestive health. Follow step-by-step instructions that transform these ingredients into delicious, nutrient-rich elixirs.

Explore the nutritional information accompanying each recipe, empowering you to make choices aligned with your well-being goals. Uncover ingredient substitutes tailored for allergies and dietary needs, ensuring that every sip is a personalized, safe indulgence.

This book is your ally in easing diverticulitis pain. Find valuable tips and tricks to soothe discomfort, allowing you to relish your juicing adventure with renewed comfort and vitality.

Finally, embrace the freedom to customize. Make these recipes uniquely yours by adding your flair. Whether it's adjusting flavors or experimenting with new ingredients, the power to make each glass your own is in your hands.

Are you ready? Let the juicing revolution begin!

JUICING DURING DIVERTICULITIS FLARE-UPS
Dos and Don'ts

Diverticulitis flare-ups can bring about discomfort and challenges when it comes to dietary choices. While juicing can be a valuable tool for digestive health, there are specific considerations to keep in mind during these periods of heightened symptoms. Here, we'll explore the dos and don'ts of juicing for diverticulitis during flare-ups to help you make informed choices for optimal well-being.

Dos:
1. Choose Low-Fiber Options:
- Opt for juicing ingredients that are gentle on the digestive system during flare-ups. Consider using peeled and deseeded fruits and well-cooked vegetables to minimize fiber content.

2. Include Soothing Ingredients:
- Incorporate ingredients known for their anti-inflammatory and soothing properties. Aloe vera, cucumber, and mint are examples of ingredients that may help alleviate inflammation and provide relief.

3. Hydrate Adequately:
- Staying hydrated is crucial during diverticulitis flare-ups. Include hydrating fruits like watermelon and incorporate coconut water to maintain fluid balance.

4. Blending Instead of Juicing:
- During flare-ups, consider blending fruits and vegetables instead of traditional juicing. Blended smoothies retain more fiber, which can be beneficial for a more gradual and gentle digestive process.

5. Seek Professional Guidance:
- They can provide guidance tailored to your specific condition, ensuring that your juicing choices align with your overall treatment plan.

Don'ts:
1. Avoid High-Fiber Ingredients:
- Steer clear of high-fiber fruits and vegetables during flare-ups. Ingredients like berries, seeds, and raw greens may exacerbate symptoms and irritate the inflamed areas.

2. Limit Citrus and Acidic Fruits:
- Citrus fruits and other acidic options may be harsh on an inflamed digestive tract. Limit the use of oranges, lemons, and grapefruits, and opt for milder alternatives like melons or pears.

3. Skip Spicy Additions:
- Spices and hot peppers can be irritating to the digestive system during flare-ups. Avoid adding spicy elements to your juices and focus on milder herbs like ginger for flavor.

4. Minimize Cruciferous Vegetables:
- Cruciferous vegetables like broccoli and cauliflower can be challenging for some during flare-ups. Consider juicing gentler options like carrots, zucchini, or spinach.

5. Refrain from Overconsumption:
- While juicing can be beneficial, avoid excessive intake during flare-ups. Overconsumption may overwhelm the digestive system and worsen symptoms.

Juicing can still be part of a diverticulitis management plan during flare-ups with careful consideration of ingredients. It's essential to prioritize soothing and low-fiber options, stay well-hydrated, and consult with healthcare professionals for personalized guidance. Remember that individual responses may vary, so it's crucial to listen to your body and make adjustments accordingly.

Addressing Common Issues with Juicing for Diverticulitis

Juicing can be a powerful ally in managing diverticulitis, offering a convenient way to obtain essential nutrients while minimizing digestive stress. However, as with any dietary approach, there are common challenges that individuals may encounter. Let's explore some of these issues and provide guidance on how to address them for a successful and supportive juicing experience.

1. Balancing Fiber Intake:
- **Issue:** Striking the right balance of fiber can be challenging, as too much or too little can impact digestive health.
- **Solution:** Gradually introduce fiber-rich fruits and vegetables, adjusting the quantity based on your body's response. Experiment with various ingredients to find the optimal mix that supports your digestive comfort.

2. Choosing Digestion-Friendly Ingredients:
- **Issue:** Some individuals may struggle with certain fruits or vegetables that are harder to digest.
- **Solution:** Prioritize easily digestible options, such as peeled and deseeded fruits, well-cooked vegetables, and incorporating ingredients with anti-inflammatory properties, like ginger or aloe vera.

3. Managing Flare-Ups:

- **Issue:** Flare-ups can complicate juicing routines, requiring modifications to avoid exacerbating symptoms.
- **Solution:** During flare-ups, consider blending instead of juicing to retain more fiber. Choose soothing ingredients like cucumber, mint, and aloe vera. Adjust your juicing plan based on the severity of symptoms and consult with healthcare professionals for personalized guidance.

4. Dealing with Taste Preferences:

- **Issue:** Some individuals may find it challenging to enjoy the taste of certain juiced combinations.
- **Solution:** Experiment with different flavor profiles and ingredients to find combinations that suit your taste buds. Adding a touch of natural sweetness from fruits like apples or a hint of citrus can enhance the overall taste.

5. Ensuring Adequate Hydration:

- **Issue**: Over Reliance on juicing without sufficient water intake may lead to dehydration.
- **Solution:** Supplement your juicing routine with ample water consumption throughout the day. Hydration is crucial for supporting digestive health and overall well-being.

6. Monitoring Portion Sizes:

- **Issue:** Consuming overly large juice portions may overwhelm the digestive system.

- **Solution**: Be mindful of portion sizes and consume juices in moderation. Smaller, more frequent servings may be gentler on the digestive tract.

7. Addressing Nutrient Gaps:
- **Issue:** Depending solely on juicing may result in nutrient gaps.
- **Solution:** Use juicing as a complement to a well-rounded diet. Incorporate a variety of whole foods to ensure you receive a broad spectrum of nutrients. Consider consulting a dietitian for personalized nutritional advice.

8. Navigating Dietary Restrictions:
- **Issue:** Individuals with dietary restrictions may find it challenging to incorporate a diverse range of juicing ingredients.
- **Solution:** Explore alternative ingredients that align with your dietary needs. There is a wide variety of fruits and vegetables to choose from, allowing for flexibility in creating juices that suit your preferences and restrictions.

Addressing common issues with juicing for diverticulitis involves a combination of thoughtful ingredient selection, mindful portion control, and adapting your approach based on individual needs and responses. By staying attuned to your body and making adjustments as needed, you can harness the benefits of juicing for optimal digestive health.

HOW TO USE THIS COOKBOOK

Welcome to "*Juicing for Diverticulitis*"! To make the most of your juicing journey, follow these steps:

1. Prepare Your Ingredients: Carefully review the ingredients list before starting to ensure you have everything you need for a successful juicing experience.

2. Step-by-Step Instructions: Follow the detailed step-by-step instructions for each recipe. Pay close attention to measurements and procedures to achieve optimal flavor and nutritional benefits.

3. Nutritional Information: Discover the health benefits of each juice with provided nutritional information. This section will guide you in making informed choices tailored to your dietary goals.

4. Allergies and Dietary Needs: Find ingredient substitutes for allergies and dietary requirements. Adapt recipes to suit your individual health needs while still enjoying the delicious flavors designed for diverticulitis-friendly juicing.

5. Soothing Diverticulitis Pain: Explore valuable tips on soothing diverticulitis pain. Incorporate ingredients and practices that may alleviate discomfort, making your juicing experience both enjoyable and supportive of your well-being.

6. Customization: Make each recipe uniquely yours by incorporating personal touches and flavor preferences. Experiment with ingredient combinations to create juices that cater to your taste while maintaining their diverticulitis-friendly nature.

Cheers to vibrant living!

DIVERTICULITIS MARVELOUS MIXOLOGY

Recipe 1: Beet Bliss Elixir

Ingredients:
- 1 medium beet
- 1 apple
- 1-inch fresh ginger root
- 1 lemon
- Water

Instructions:
1. Wash and peel the beet, apple, and ginger.
2. Cut the beet, apple, and ginger into small pieces.
3. Juice the beet, apple, and ginger together.
4. Squeeze the lemon into the juice.
5. Dilute with water to desired consistency.
6. Stir well and serve chilled.

Nutritional Information:
- Beets are rich in fiber, folate, and antioxidants.
- Apples provide vitamins and minerals like vitamin C and potassium.
- Ginger has anti-inflammatory properties and aids digestion.
- Lemons contains lots of vitamin C.

Ingredient Substitutes:
- If sensitive to beets, substitute with carrots for a similar color and nutrient profile.
- Replace apple with pear for a slightly different flavor.
- Use turmeric instead of ginger for an earthy twist.

Tips for Soothing Diverticulitis:
- Beets are known to support digestive health due to their fiber content.
- Ginger can help reduce inflammation in the digestive tract.
- Apples provide soluble fiber that aids digestion.

Recipe 2: Ginger Zest Infusion

Ingredients:
- Fresh ginger
- Honey
- Lemon
- Water
- Organic flavors (optional)

Instructions:
1. Peel and slice the fresh ginger into thin rounds.
2. Boil water in a pot and add the ginger slices.
3. Let the ginger simmer in water for 10-15 minutes to infuse its flavor.
4. Remove the pot from heat and add honey to taste.
5. Squeeze fresh lemon juice into the mixture.
6. Strain the infusion to remove ginger pieces.
7. Serve hot or chilled over ice.

Nutritional Information:
- Ginger aids digestion and is known for its anti-inflammatory properties.
- Honey provides natural sweetness and may have antibacterial properties.
- Lemon adds a refreshing citrus flavor and is rich in vitamin C.

Ingredient Substitutes:
- Substitute maple syrup with honey for a vegan option.
- Replace lemon with orange for a different citrus twist.
- Add a cinnamon stick for additional flavor and warmth.

Tips for Soothing Diverticulitis:
- Ginger can help reduce inflammation in the digestive tract, aiding in soothing diverticulitis symptoms.
- Lemon adds a refreshing touch and may assist in digestion.
- Honey provides a natural sweetness without added sugars that can irritate the digestive system.

Recipe 3: Apple Spinach Serenity

Ingredients:
- 2 apples
- 2 cups spinach
- 4-5 carrots
- Honey (optional)
- Water

Instructions:
1. Wash all the fruits and vegetables thoroughly.
2. Peel and core the apples, then cut them into chunks.
3. Cut the carrots into pieces suitable for juicing.
4. Add spinach, apples, and carrots to the juicer.
5. Juice the ingredients together.
6. Sweeten with honey if desired.
7. Serve immediately over ice.

Nutritional Information:
- Apples provide vitamins and fiber.
- Spinach is rich in B vitamins, vitamins A, C, and K.
- Carrots offer beta-carotene and essential minerals.

Ingredient Substitutes:
- Substitute pears for apples for a slightly different flavor.
- Use kale instead of spinach for a nutrient-rich alternative.
- Agave syrup can replace honey for a vegan option.

Tips for Soothing Diverticulitis:
- Spinach and carrots are gentle on the digestive system and provide essential nutrients.
- Apples add natural sweetness without overwhelming the digestive tract.

Recipe 4: Pineapple Cucumber Quencher

Ingredients:
- 1 cup pineapple chunks
- 1 cucumber
- Mint leaves
- Lime
- Water

Instructions:
1. Peel and chop the cucumber into chunks.
2. Cut the pineapple into small pieces.
3. Blend cucumber, pineapple, and a handful of mint leaves with water.
4. Squeeze fresh lime juice into the mixture.
5. Blend until smooth.
6. Strain if desired or serve as is over ice.

Nutritional Information:
- Pineapple is rich in vitamin C and manganese.
- Cucumber provides hydration and a refreshing taste.
- Mint helps improve digestion and adds a fresh flavor.

Ingredient Substitutes:
- Replace mint with basil for a different herbal note.
- Lemon can be used instead of lime for a citrus variation.
- Add a splash of coconut water for extra hydration.

Tips for Soothing Diverticulitis:
- Pineapple contains bromelain, an enzyme that may help with digestion.
- Cucumber is hydrating and gentle on the stomach, aiding in soothing diverticulitis symptoms.

SOOTHING SIPS SERENADE
Recipe 5: Carrot Ginger Soothe

Ingredients:
- 4-5 carrots
- 1-inch fresh ginger
- Honey (optional)
- Water
- Lemon

Instructions:
1. Wash and peel the carrots and ginger.
2. Cut the carrots into pieces suitable for juicing.
3. Peel and slice the ginger into small chunks.
4. Juice the carrots and ginger together.
5. Squeeze fresh lemon juice into the mixture.
6. Sweeten with honey if desired.
7. Dilute with water to desired consistency.
8. Stir well and serve chilled.

Nutritional Information:
- Carrots are rich in beta-carotene and fiber.
- Ginger helps improve digestion and has anti-inflammatory properties.
- Lemon provides vitamin C and adds a refreshing touch.

Ingredient Substitutes:
- Use turmeric instead of ginger for a different flavor profile.
- Agave syrup can replace honey for a vegan option.

- Lime juice can be used instead of lemon for a citrus variation.

Tips for Soothing Diverticulitis:
- Carrots are gentle on the digestive system and provide essential nutrients.
- Ginger can help reduce inflammation in the digestive tract, aiding in soothing diverticulitis symptoms.

Recipe 6: Cucumber Melon Chill

Ingredients:
- 1 cucumber
- 1/2 honeydew melon
- Mint leaves
- Lime
- Water

Instructions:
1. Peel and chop the cucumber into chunks.
2. Remove seeds from the honeydew melon and cut into pieces.
3. Blend cucumber, honeydew melon, and a handful of mint leaves with water.
4. Squeeze fresh lime juice into the mixture.
5. Blend until smooth.
6. Strain if desired or serve as is over ice.

Nutritional Information:
- Cucumber provides hydration and a refreshing taste.
- Honeydew melon is rich in vitamins C and K, as well as antioxidants.
- Mint helps improve digestion and adds a fresh flavor.

Ingredient Substitutes:
- Replace honeydew melon with cantaloupe for a similar taste profile.
- Lemon can be used instead of lime for a citrus variation.

- Basil leaves can be used instead of mint for a different herbal note.

Tips for Soothing Diverticulitis:
- Cucumber is hydrating and gentle on the stomach, aiding in soothing diverticulitis symptoms.
- Honeydew melon provides essential vitamins while being easy to digest.

Recipe 7: Soothing Chamomile Dream

Ingredients:
- 1 cup boiling water
- 1 chamomile tea bag
- Honey (optional)

Instructions:
1. In a kettle or pot boil water.
2. Place the chamomile tea bag in a cup or mug.
3. Slowly pour the boiling water over the tea bag.
4. Steep for about 3-5 minutes, depending on desired strength.
5. Remove the tea bag and add honey to taste, if desired.
6. Enjoy warm or cold.

Nutritional Information:
- Chamomile tea is caffeine-free and has calming properties.
- Honey provides natural sweetness and may have antibacterial properties.

Ingredient Substitutes:
- Use peppermint tea for a slightly different flavor profile.
- Agave syrup can replace honey for a vegan option.
- Add a splash of vanilla extract for an additional aromatic touch.

Tips for Soothing Diverticulitis:
- Chamomile tea is popular for its anti-inflammatory properties, which can help soothe the digestive system.
- Honey provides a natural sweetness without overwhelming the digestive tract.

Recipe 8: Calming Lavender Tranquili-Tea

Ingredients:
- 1 cup boiling water
- 1 lavender tea bag
- Honey (optional)

Instructions:
1. In a kettle or pot boil water
2. Place the lavender tea bag in a cup or mug.
3. Pour the boiling water over the tea bag.
4. Steep for about 3-5 minutes, depending on desired strength.
5. Remove the tea bag and add honey to taste, if desired.
6. Enjoy warm or cold.

Nutritional Information:
- Lavender tea has a calming effect and may aid in relaxation.
- Honey provides natural sweetness and may have antibacterial properties.

Ingredient Substitutes:
- Use chamomile tea for a similar flavor profile.
- Substitute maple syrup with honey for a vegan option.
- Add a splash of lemon juice for a refreshing twist.

Tips for Soothing Diverticulitis:
- Lavender tea has a calming effect on the digestive system, which can help soothe diverticulitis symptoms.
- Honey provides a natural sweetness without overwhelming the digestive tract.

VIBRANT VITALITY REVIVAL RENDEZVOUS

Recipe 9: Mint Cucumber Cooler Juice

Ingredients:
- 1 cucumber
- 10 fresh mint leaves
- 1 cup water

Instructions:
1. Juice the cucumber in a juicer.
2. Blend the mint leaves with water in a blender.
3. Combine the cucumber juice and mint-water blend.
4. Serve chilled for a refreshing drink.

Nutritional Information:
- Cucumber provides hydration and essential minerals.
- Mint adds a cooling sensation and may aid in digestion.

Ingredient Substitutes:
- Use a different herb like basil or parsley for a different flavor.
- Replace cucumber with a different vegetable like celery or carrot.

Tips:
- This juice can be enjoyed as a refreshing drink during a clear liquid diet for diverticulitis.
- It is essential to consult with your healthcare provider before incorporating new juices into your diet to ensure they are suitable for your specific needs and dietary restrictions.

Recipe 10: Strawberry Banana Delight Juice

Ingredients:
- 1 Banana, sliced
- 1 cup Frozen strawberries
- 1 cup Milk of choice
- 1/2 cup Water
- 3-4 Ice cubes

Instructions:
1. Combine the sliced banana, frozen strawberries, milk, water, and ice cubes in a blender.
2. Blend the ingredients until smooth and well mixed.
3. Pour the juice into a glass.
4. Garnish with fresh strawberry slices if desired.
5. Serve chilled and enjoy this delightful Strawberry Banana juice.

Nutritional Information:
- Bananas provide potassium and fiber.
- Strawberries are rich in vitamin C and antioxidants.
- Milk adds calcium and protein to the juice.

Ingredient Substitutes:
- Use almond milk or coconut milk as a dairy-free alternative.
- Substitute frozen strawberries with fresh ones if preferred.

Tips for Soothing Diverticulitis:
- This Strawberry Banana Delight Juice offers a blend of soothing flavors and nutrients that can be gentle on the digestive system during diverticulitis flare-ups.
- Ensure the ingredients are well blended to avoid any large pieces that may be difficult to digest.
- Adjust the consistency by adding more water or ice cubes for a lighter drink.

Recipe 11: Pear-fectly Rejuvenate

Ingredients:
- 2 ripe pears
- 1 cup spinach
- 1/2 cucumber
- 1/2 lemon
- 1/2 inch ginger
- 1 cup water

Instructions:
1. Peel and core the pears.
2. Wash and prepare the spinach, cucumber, and ginger.
3. Juice the pears, spinach, cucumber, and ginger.
4. Squeeze the juice from the lemon.
5. Combine the pear juice, spinach juice, cucumber juice, ginger juice, and lemon juice in a blender.
6. Add water to the blender and blend until smooth.
7. Pour the mixture into a glass and serve immediately.

Nutritional Information:
- Pears are rich in fiber and vitamins C and K.
- Spinach is high in iron and vitamins A, C, and K.
- Cucumber provides hydration and antioxidants.
- Lemon adds vitamin C and a refreshing taste.
- Ginger helps improve digestion and has anti-inflammatory properties.

Ingredient Substitutes:
- Use apples instead of pears for a similar taste profile.
- Replace the spinach with kale for a slightly different flavor and nutrient profile.
- Substitute cucumber with celery for a milder taste.

Tips for Soothing Diverticulitis:
- This pear-based juice provides essential nutrients that can aid in soothing diverticulitis symptoms.
- The combination of fruits and vegetables offers fiber, vitamins, and minerals that are beneficial for digestive health.

Recipe 12: Ginger Lemon Detox Juice

Ingredients:
- 1/2 lemon, juiced
- 1/2 inch knob of ginger root, grated
- 12 ounces water at room temperature

Instructions:
1. Juice the lemon and grate the ginger into a glass.
2. Add the grated ginger to the glass of water.
3. Stir the ingredients together.
4. Serve chilled for a refreshing and detoxifying drink.

Nutritional Information:
- Lemon provides vitamin C and aids in digestion.
- Ginger boosts metabolism and helps improve digestion.

Ingredient Substitutes:
- Substitute lime juice with lemon for a different flavor.
- Replace ginger with turmeric for an anti-inflammatory boost.

Tips:
- This Ginger Lemon Detox Juice can be incorporated into a 3-day cleanse or enjoyed as a daily detox drink.
- Drink this juice first thing in the morning to kickstart your metabolism and flush out toxins.

TROPICAL TEMPTATIONS BLISS BASH

Recipe 13: Coconut Lime Refresher Juice

Ingredients:
- 2 cups Coconut water
- 1/4-1/2 cup Canned coconut milk or cream
- 1-2 Tbsp Fresh lime juice (approximately 1 lime)
- Ice for serving

Instructions:
1. In a blender, combine the coconut water, canned coconut milk, and fresh lime juice.
2. Blend the ingredients until well combined.
3. Adjust the taste by adding more coconut milk for creaminess, more lime juice for tanginess, or more coconut water for sweetness.
4. Pour the mixture into glasses filled with ice.
5. Garnish with a lime wedge if desired.
6. Enjoy this refreshing Coconut Lime Refresher.

Nutritional Information:
- Coconut water provides hydration and electrolytes.
- Canned coconut milk adds creaminess and richness.
- Lime juice offers a tangy flavor and vitamin C.

Ingredient Substitutes:
- Substitute fresh lime juice with lemon juice for a different citrus twist.
- Opt for light coconut milk for a lower-calorie option.

Tips for Soothing Diverticulitis:
- This Coconut Lime Refresher is a hydrating and refreshing drink that can be soothing for individuals with diverticulitis.

- Adjust the sweetness by adding a natural sweetener like honey or agave syrup to suit your taste (optional).

Recipe 14: Sunset Slush Sensation:

Ingredients:
- 2 cups frozen strawberries
- 1 cup orange juice
- 1/2 cup pineapple juice
- 1/4 cup honey
- Ice cubes

Instructions:
1. In a blender, combine frozen strawberries, orange juice, pineapple juice, and honey.
2. Add ice cubes to the blender for a slushier consistency.
3. Blend until smooth and well combined.
4. Pour the slush into glasses and serve immediately.

Nutritional Information:
- Strawberries are rich in vitamin C and antioxidants.
- Orange juice provides vitamin C and natural sweetness.
- Pineapple juice adds tropical flavor and vitamin C.
- Honey offers natural sweetness and potential health benefits.

Ingredient Substitutes:
- Use frozen mixed berries instead of just strawberries for a variety of flavors.
- Substitute apple juice for orange juice for a different fruity taste.
- Replace honey with agave syrup for a vegan alternative.

Tips for Soothing Diverticulitis:
- This fruity slush sensation can be a refreshing treat that is gentle on the digestive system.
- The combination of fruits in this slush provides vitamins and antioxidants that can support digestive health.

Recipe 15: Hydrating Electrolyte Elixir

Ingredients:
- 1 cup water
- 1/4 cup lemon juice
- 1/4 cup lime juice
- 1/4 cup orange juice
- 1/4 cup apple juice
- 1/4 cup pineapple juice
- 1/4 cup coconut water
- 1/4 cup honey (optional)

Instructions:
1. Combine water, lemon juice, lime juice, orange juice, apple juice, pineapple juice, and coconut water in a blender.
2. Blend the ingredients until smooth and well mixed.
3. Add honey to sweeten the elixir (optional).
4. Pour the mixture into a glass and enjoy.

Nutritional Information:
- Water provides hydration and no calories.
- Lemon juice adds vitamin C and a tart flavor.
- Lime juice offers vitamin C and a tangy taste.
- Orange juice provides vitamin C and natural sweetness.
- Apple juice contributes vitamin C and a mild sweetness.
- Pineapple juice adds bromelain, which can help with digestion and vitamin C.
- Coconut water offers electrolytes and hydration.

Ingredient Substitutes:
- Use a different fruit juice, such as grapefruit or cranberry, for a different flavor profile.
- Substitute honey with agave syrup or another natural sweetener for a vegan alternative.
- Replace coconut water with another clear liquid, such as water or clear broth, for a non-alcoholic version.

Tips for Soothing Diverticulitis:
- This hydrating electrolyte elixir is designed to be gentle on the digestive system during a diverticulitis flare-up.
- The combination of fruits and coconut water provides essential nutrients and electrolytes that can support the body's natural healing process.
- It is essential to consult with your healthcare provider before incorporating this juice into your diet to ensure it is appropriate for your specific needs and dietary restrictions.

Recipe 16: Mango Mint Delight Juice

Ingredients:
- 1 ½ cups frozen mango (or 1 fresh mango)
- 1 carrot
- 1 tablespoon desiccated coconut
- Pulp of 1 passionfruit
- Handful of mint leaves

Instructions:
1. If using fresh mango, peel and chop it into chunks.
2. Peel and chop the carrot.
3. In a blender, combine the frozen or fresh mango, carrot, desiccated coconut, passionfruit pulp, and mint leaves.
4. Blend until smooth and well combined.
5. Strain the juice if desired for a smoother texture.
6. Serve chilled over ice for a delightful and refreshing drink.

Nutritional Information:
- Mango provides vitamin C and antioxidants.
- Carrots offer beta-carotene and fiber.
- Mint adds a refreshing flavor and may aid in digestion.

Ingredient Substitutes:
- Substitute desiccated coconut with coconut milk for added creaminess.
- Use pineapple instead of mango for a tropical twist.

Tips for Soothing Diverticulitis:

- This Mango Mint Delight Juice is rich in nutrients and flavors that can be soothing for individuals with diverticulitis.

- Adjust the sweetness by adding a natural sweetener like honey or agave syrup (optional).

CLEAR COMFORT CREATIONS
Recipe 17: Papaya Turmeric Lemonade

Ingredients:
- 1 cup sugar
- 1 cup boiling water
- 3 1/2 cups cold water, divided
- 3 cups peeled chopped papayas
- 1 cup fresh lemon juice (4 large lemons)

Instructions:
1. Combine sugar and boiling water in a pitcher, stirring until the sugar dissolves.
2. Allow the sugar syrup to cool slightly.
3. In a blender, combine the sugar syrup, 2 cups of cold water, chopped papayas, and fresh lemon juice.
4. Blend until the mixture is smooth.
5. Stir in the remaining 1 1/2 cups of cold water.
6. Serve the Papaya Turmeric Lemonade over ice for a refreshing drink.

Nutritional Information:
- Papayas are rich in antioxidants, vitamin C, and fiber.
- Lemon juice provides vitamin C and helps improve digestion.

Ingredient Substitutes:
- Substitute part of the sugar with a natural sweetener like honey or agave syrup for a healthier option.

- Add a pinch of ground turmeric to the lemonade for an anti-inflammatory boost.

Tips:

- This Papaya Turmeric Lemonade is a refreshing and hydrating drink that can be soothing for individuals with diverticulitis.

- Adjust the sweetness by reducing the amount of sugar used or adding more lemon juice for a tangier flavor.

Recipe 18: Cucumber Kiwi Kale Juice

Ingredients:
- 1 kiwi, peeled
- 1 medium cucumber
- 4 large leaves of kale
- 1 lemon, juiced

Instructions:
1. Wash the kiwi, cucumber, and kale thoroughly.
2. Peel the kiwi and chop it into chunks.
3. Chop the cucumber into smaller pieces.
4. Remove the stems from the kale leaves.
5. In a blender, combine the kiwi, cucumber, kale leaves, and lemon juice.
6. Blend until smooth and well combined.
7. Strain the juice if desired for a smoother texture.
8. Serve the Cucumber Kiwi Kale Juice immediately for a refreshing drink.

Nutritional Information:
- Kiwi provides vitamin C and fiber.
- Cucumber offers hydration and essential minerals.
- Kale contains lots of vitamins A, C, and K.
- Lemon juice adds a tangy flavor and vitamin C.

Ingredient Substitutes:
- Substitute lemon with lime for a slightly different citrus flavor.
- Use spinach instead of kale for a milder taste.

Tips for Soothing Diverticulitis:

- This Cucumber Kiwi Kale Juice is packed with nutrients that can be soothing for individuals with diverticulitis.

- Adjust the sweetness by adding a natural sweetener like honey or agave syrup (optional).

Recipe 19: Apple Cinnamon Cozy Tea

Ingredients:
- 2 cups filtered water
- ½ cup unfiltered fresh pressed apple cider or apple juice
- 2 Ceylon cinnamon sticks
- 1 teaspoon whole cloves
- 1 star anise

Instructions:
1. In a saucepan, combine water, apple cider, cinnamon sticks, cloves, and star anise.
2. Simmer the mixture for about 10 minutes to infuse the flavors.
3. Remove from heat and strain the tea to remove the spices.
4. Sweeten with honey or maple syrup if desired.
5. Serve hot and enjoy the cozy apple cinnamon tea.

Nutritional Information:
- Apple cider provides natural sweetness and vitamin C.
- Cinnamon offers a warm and comforting flavor along with potential health benefits.
- Cloves and star anise add aromatic notes and may have digestive benefits.

Ingredient Substitutes:
- Use apple juice instead of apple cider for a slightly different taste.
- Substitute whole cloves with ground cloves if whole cloves are not available.

- Replace star anise with a pinch of nutmeg or allspice for a different spice profile.

Tips for Soothing Diverticulitis:
- This Apple Cinnamon Cozy Tea can be soothing for diverticulitis due to its gentle flavors and warmth.
- The combination of apple and cinnamon provides a comforting drink that can help relax the digestive system.
- It is advisable to consult with your healthcare provider before adding this tea to your diet to ensure it aligns with your specific dietary needs during diverticulitis management.

Recipe 20: Soothing Ginger Soother:

Ingredients:
- 2 gala apples, thinly sliced
- 5-7 thinly sliced ginger pieces
- 2 whole cinnamon sticks
- 2 tablespoons pure maple syrup
- 4 ½ cups water

Instructions:
1. Place all the ingredients in a large pot and cook on medium-low heat for one hour.
2. Strain the liquid through a strainer or mesh cloth.
3. Transfer the tea to a kettle or ladle it directly into a teacup.

Recipe Variations:
- During the holidays, substitute water with orange juice and add a few whole cloves.
- This recipe can be doubled or tripled; ensure you use a large enough pot.
- Use a slow cooker on low heat for 2-3 hours or high heat for 1-2 hours.

Nutritional Information:
- Apple Cinnamon Tea is rich in Vitamin C from apples and antioxidants from cinnamon.
- It may help improve blood sugar levels and provide soothing relief, especially for sore throats.

TROUBLESHOOTING TIPS FOR A SUCCESSFUL JUICING JOURNEY

Starting a juicing journey for digestive health is a commendable step towards wellness. However, like any adventure, challenges may arise along the way. Whether you're new to juicing or looking to refine your approach, here are some troubleshooting tips to help you overcome common hurdles and make your juicing experience both enjoyable and effective.

1. Issue: Bitter Taste in Juices:
- **Solution:** Counteract bitterness with naturally sweet fruits like apples, pineapples, or berries. Add a hint of citrus for a refreshing twist. Experiment with different fruit combinations to find a balance that suits your taste buds.

2. Issue: Separation of Juice Components:
- **Solution:** Natural separation is normal. To combat this, stir your juice before consuming or consider using a juicer with slower rotation to minimize separation. Adding ingredients like chia seeds or blending instead of juicing can also enhance consistency.

3. Issue: Difficulty Cleaning the Juicer:
- **Solution:** Clean your juicer immediately after use to prevent residue buildup. Disassemble parts for thorough cleaning and use a brush for hard-to-reach areas. Refer to your juicer's manual for specific cleaning instructions.

4. Issue: Overloading on High-Sugar Ingredients:
- **Solution**: While fruits add sweetness, overloading on high-sugar fruits can impact blood sugar levels. Balance sweetness with vegetables like cucumber or celery. Experiment with lower-sugar fruits like berries or opt for green juices with minimal fruit content.

5. Issue: Digestive Discomfort:
- **Solution**: Introduce fiber gradually to avoid digestive discomfort. Peel and deseed fruits and opt for well-cooked vegetables. Include soothing ingredients like aloe vera or mint to support digestive health. If the discomfort doesn't stop, consult with a healthcare professional immediately.

6. Issue: Lack of Variety:
- **Solution**: Include different fruits and vegetables to ensure a broad spectrum of nutrients. Rotate your ingredients weekly to keep your taste buds engaged and maximize nutritional benefits.

7. Issue: Budget Constraints:
- **Solution:** Juicing can be cost-effective with strategic choices. Purchase seasonal produce, buy in bulk, and explore local farmers' markets for budget-friendly options. Consider frozen fruits and vegetables as a convenient substitute.

8. Issue: Inconsistent Texture:
- **Solution:** Achieve consistent texture by blending or processing ingredients in batches. Choose fruits and vegetables with similar textures for a smoother juice. Experiment with combinations to find a texture that suits your preference.

9. Issue: Foamy Juices:
- **Solution:** Foamy juices are common, especially with certain fruits. Let your juice settle for a few minutes before consuming, or use a fine mesh strainer to reduce foam. Adding ingredients like cucumber or celery can also minimize foaming.

10. Issue: Lack of Time:
- **Solution:** Plan and prepare ingredients in advance to streamline your juicing process. Consider batch juicing for multiple servings and store them in airtight containers in the fridge. Set a regular juicing schedule to make it a consistent part of your routine.

By addressing these common challenges with practical solutions, you can navigate your juicing journey more smoothly and derive maximum benefits for your digestive health. Remember, juicing is a personal experience, so feel free to adapt these tips to suit your preferences and lifestyle. Happy juicing!

CONCLUSION

As you close the pages of "Juicing for Diverticulitis" by Aveline Winter, remember that your journey towards digestive well-being is an ongoing adventure. Through vibrant concoctions and thoughtful guidance, we've explored the world of juicing as a flavorful remedy for diverticulitis.

I hope this book has not only equipped you with the tools to create delicious, nutritious juices but also inspired a deeper connection with your well-being. Your health is a journey, and each sip is a step towards a more vibrant, comfortable life.

As you savor the unique blends, remember the power lies within you to customize, adapt, and make each recipe your own. Let your creativity flow as you embrace the joy of personalizing your juicing experience.

May this book be a constant companion on your path to digestive harmony. Here's to a future filled with wellness, flavor, and the delightful embrace of "*Juicing for Diverticulitis.*"

Cheers to your health and the countless glasses of vitality that await you!

Juicing planner

MONDAY **TUESDAY** **WEDNESDAY**

THURSDAY **FRIDAY** **SHOPPING LIST**

SATURDAY **SUNDAY**

notes

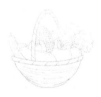

Juicing planner

MONDAY	TUESDAY	WEDNESDAY

THURSDAY	FRIDAY	SHOPPING LIST

SATURDAY	SUNDAY

notes

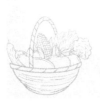

Juicing planner

MONDAY	TUESDAY	WEDNESDAY

THURSDAY	FRIDAY	SHOPPING LIST

SATURDAY	SUNDAY

notes

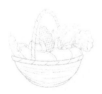

Juicing planner

MONDAY	TUESDAY	WEDNESDAY

THURSDAY	FRIDAY	SHOPPING LIST

SATURDAY	SUNDAY

Notes

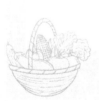

Juicing planner

MONDAY	TUESDAY	WEDNESDAY

THURSDAY	FRIDAY	SHOPPING LIST

SATURDAY	SUNDAY	

notes

Juicing planner

MONDAY	TUESDAY	WEDNESDAY

THURSDAY	FRIDAY	SHOPPING LIST

SATURDAY	SUNDAY

notes

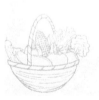

Juicing planner

MONDAY	TUESDAY	WEDNESDAY

THURSDAY	FRIDAY	SHOPPING LIST

SATURDAY	SUNDAY

notes

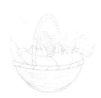

Juicing planner

MONDAY	TUESDAY	WEDNESDAY

THURSDAY	FRIDAY	SHOPPING LIST

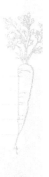

SATURDAY	SUNDAY

Notes

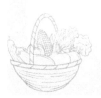

Juicing planner

MONDAY   TUESDAY   WEDNESDAY

THURSDAY   FRIDAY   SHOPPING LIST

SATURDAY   SUNDAY

 notes

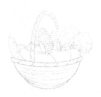

Juicing planner

MONDAY	TUESDAY	WEDNESDAY

THURSDAY	FRIDAY	SHOPPING LIST

SATURDAY	SUNDAY

notes

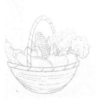

Juicing planner

MONDAY   TUESDAY   WEDNESDAY

THURSDAY   FRIDAY   SHOPPING LIST

SATURDAY   SUNDAY

notes

Juicing planner

MONDAY	TUESDAY	WEDNESDAY

THURSDAY	FRIDAY	SHOPPING LIST

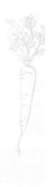

SATURDAY	SUNDAY	

notes

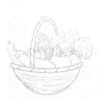

Juicing planner

MONDAY	TUESDAY	WEDNESDAY

THURSDAY	FRIDAY	SHOPPING LIST

SATURDAY	SUNDAY

Notes

Juicing planner

MONDAY	TUESDAY	WEDNESDAY

THURSDAY	FRIDAY	SHOPPING LIST

SATURDAY	SUNDAY

notes

Juicing planner

MONDAY	TUESDAY	WEDNESDAY

THURSDAY	FRIDAY	SHOPPING LIST

SATURDAY	SUNDAY

notes

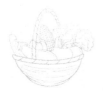

Juicing planner

MONDAY	TUESDAY	WEDNESDAY

THURSDAY	FRIDAY	SHOPPING LIST

SATURDAY	SUNDAY

notes

Juicing planner

MONDAY

TUESDAY

WEDNESDAY

THURSDAY

FRIDAY

SHOPPING LIST

SATURDAY

SUNDAY

Notes

Juicing planner

MONDAY	TUESDAY	WEDNESDAY

THURSDAY	FRIDAY	SHOPPING LIST

SATURDAY	SUNDAY

notes

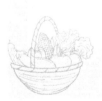

Juicing planner

MONDAY	TUESDAY	WEDNESDAY

THURSDAY	FRIDAY	SHOPPING LIST

SATURDAY	SUNDAY

 notes

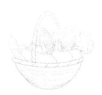

Juicing planner

MONDAY	TUESDAY	WEDNESDAY

THURSDAY	FRIDAY	SHOPPING LIST

SATURDAY	SUNDAY

notes

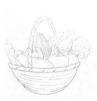

Juicing planner

MONDAY	TUESDAY	WEDNESDAY

THURSDAY	FRIDAY	SHOPPING LIST

SATURDAY	SUNDAY

notes

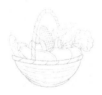

Juicing planner

MONDAY	TUESDAY	WEDNESDAY

THURSDAY	FRIDAY	SHOPPING LIST

SATURDAY	SUNDAY

Notes

Juicing planner

MONDAY	TUESDAY	WEDNESDAY

THURSDAY	FRIDAY	SHOPPING LIST

SATURDAY	SUNDAY

notes

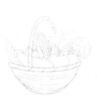

Juicing planner

MONDAY TUESDAY WEDNESDAY

THURSDAY FRIDAY SHOPPING LIST

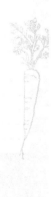

SATURDAY SUNDAY

notes

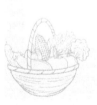

Juicing planner

MONDAY	TUESDAY	WEDNESDAY

THURSDAY	FRIDAY	SHOPPING LIST

SATURDAY	SUNDAY

notes

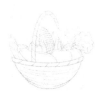

Juicing planner

MONDAY	TUESDAY	WEDNESDAY

THURSDAY	FRIDAY	SHOPPING LIST

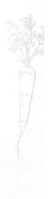

SATURDAY	SUNDAY

Notes

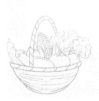

Juicing planner

MONDAY	TUESDAY	WEDNESDAY

THURSDAY	FRIDAY	SHOPPING LIST

SATURDAY	SUNDAY

notes

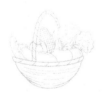

Juicing planner

MONDAY	TUESDAY	WEDNESDAY

THURSDAY	FRIDAY	SHOPPING LIST

SATURDAY	SUNDAY

notes

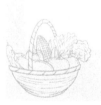

Juicing planner

MONDAY   TUESDAY   WEDNESDAY

THURSDAY   FRIDAY   SHOPPING LIST

SATURDAY   SUNDAY

Notes

Juicing planner

MONDAY	TUESDAY	WEDNESDAY

THURSDAY	FRIDAY	SHOPPING LIST

SATURDAY	SUNDAY

Notes

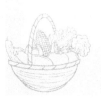

A HEARTFELT THANK YOU!

Thank you for your support on this culinary journey! If you enjoyed this book, please consider creating a video review or, if that's not feasible, leaving a written review. You can include a picture of the book or a page that caught your interest.

STEPS ON HOW TO LEAVE A REVIEW FOR THIS BOOK

1. Scan the QR code with your phone camera, a link will pop up on your screen, simply click on it to visit my author page.

2. Scroll down and locate the book titled "JUICING FOR DIVERTICULITIS" by Aveline Winter.

3. Once you find the book, click on its title to navigate to the book's sales page.

4. Scroll down on the sales page, and right after the "About the Author" section, you'll find the "Customer Reviews" section.

5. In the "Customer Reviews" section, you'll see an option to leave a review. Begin by rating the book with stars, indicating your overall satisfaction with it.

6. After rating, a text box or prompt will appear for you to leave a written review. Share your thoughts, experiences, and any feedback you have about the book.

7. Once you've written your review, double-check to ensure everything looks good, and then submit your review.

Your feedback is invaluable and greatly appreciated!
Thank you for taking the time to share your thoughts on
"JUICING FOR DIVERTICULITIS "

Made in the USA
Las Vegas, NV
02 May 2024

89438910R00049